AF228943

DEALING WITH ADDICTION

SOCIAL MEDIA ADDICTION

by Marie-Therese Miller, PhD

BrightPoint Press

San Diego, CA

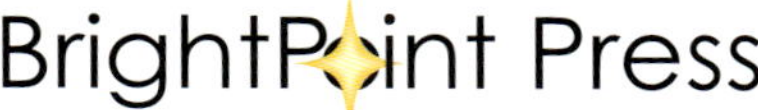

Content Consultant: Ann Liao, PhD, Associate Professor of Communication, Buffalo State College, State University of New York

LIBRARY OF CONGRESS CATALOGING-IN-PUBLICATION DATA

Names: Miller, Marie-Therese, author.
Title: Social media addiction / by Marie-Therese Miller.
Description: San Diego, CA: BrightPoint Press, [2023] | Series: Dealing
   with addiction | Includes bibliographical references and index. |
   Audience: Grades 10-12
Identifiers: LCCN 2022008623 (print) | LCCN 2022008624 (eBook) | ISBN
   9781678203788 (hardcover) | ISBN 9781678203795 (pdf)
Subjects: LCSH: Social media addiction--Juvenile literature.
Classification: LCC RC569.5.I54 M55 2023 (print) | LCC RC569.5.I54
   (eBook) | DDC 616.85/84--dc23/eng/20220309
LC record available at https://lccn.loc.gov/2022008623
LC eBook record available at https://lccn.loc.gov/2022008624

CONTENTS

- Social media sites are online services or apps that allow people to interact. Some examples include Facebook, Instagram, Reddit, and TikTok.

- Some people use social media too much. It interferes with their lives. This is called problematic social media use.

- Some experts call problematic social media use social media addiction. But the American Psychiatric Association does not consider it an addiction.

- People with problematic social media use constantly think about social media. They can't stop using it even when it negatively affects their lives.

- Using social media can release the chemical dopamine into the brain. Dopamine makes people feel good.

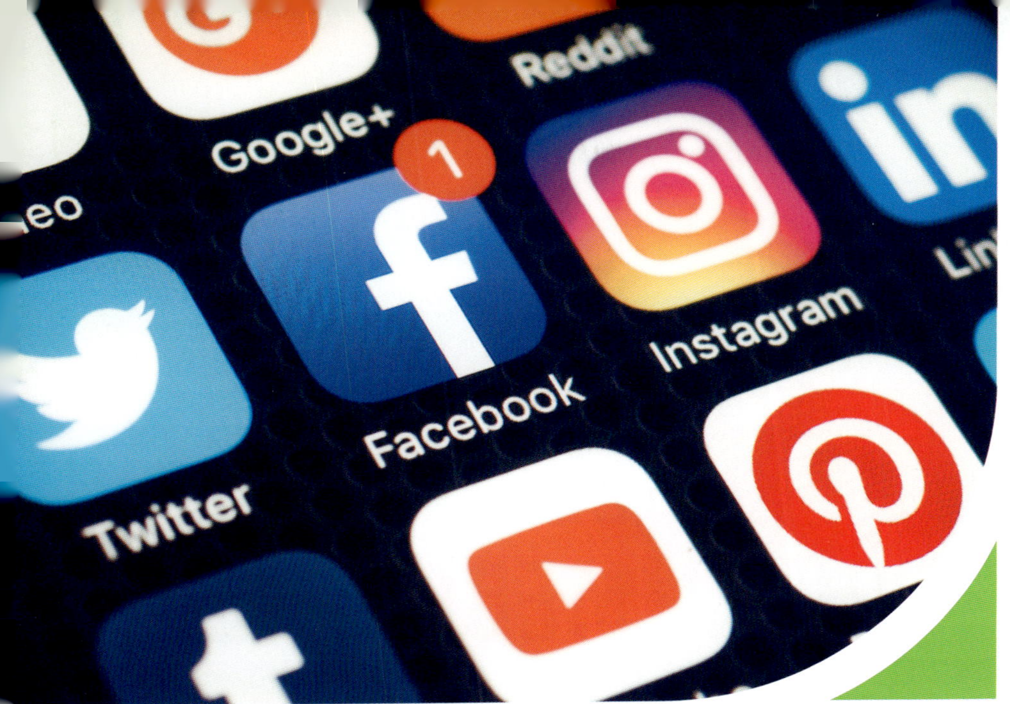

- Social media gives users positive social rewards, such as likes and kind comments. These rewards keep users coming back to the site or app.

- Problematic social media use is linked to physical and mental health disorders. Social media overuse can interfere with relationships.

- There are treatments for problematic social media use. Talk therapy is one example.

- People with problematic social media use must learn healthy ways to use technology.

LIVING WITH PROBLEMATIC SOCIAL MEDIA USE

Maya loves social media. She scrolls through her feed for hours. She snaps photos of her food and sunsets. Then she shares them on Instagram. She constantly checks how many likes the pictures get. It makes her feel good when followers like her photos.

Maya even takes her smartphone to bed. She often stays up late on social media. In the morning, she checks it before she gets up. When Maya isn't on social media, she is thinking about it. She wonders what photo to share next.

People with problematic social media use may spend a lot of time planning their posts.

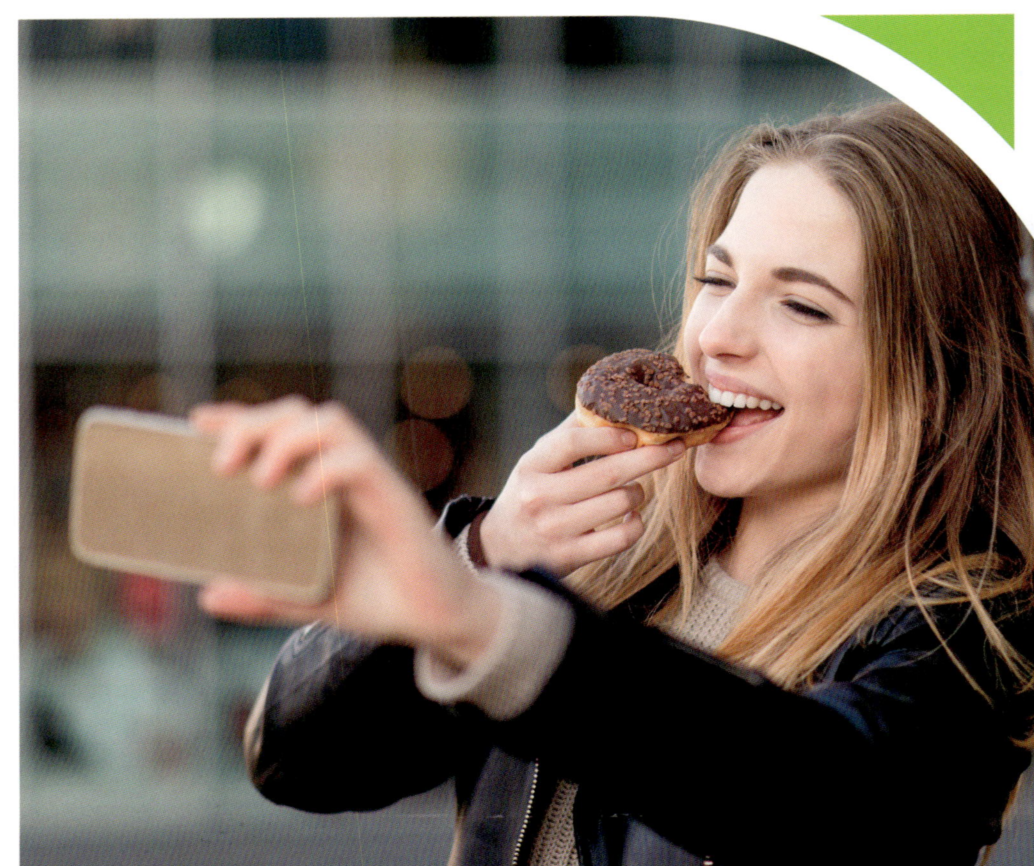

Maya doesn't feel physically or mentally healthy. She is often tired. She is out of shape because she doesn't exercise.

Her friends invite her to go out. But Maya chooses to stay home and be online. She is losing her real-life friends. Maya feels lonely.

Maya spends time on social media instead of doing her schoolwork. Her grades are dropping. Maya's parents are worried about the time she gives to social media. They often argue with her about it.

Maya is dealing with problematic social media use. Some people call it social media addiction. Maya decides to visit a

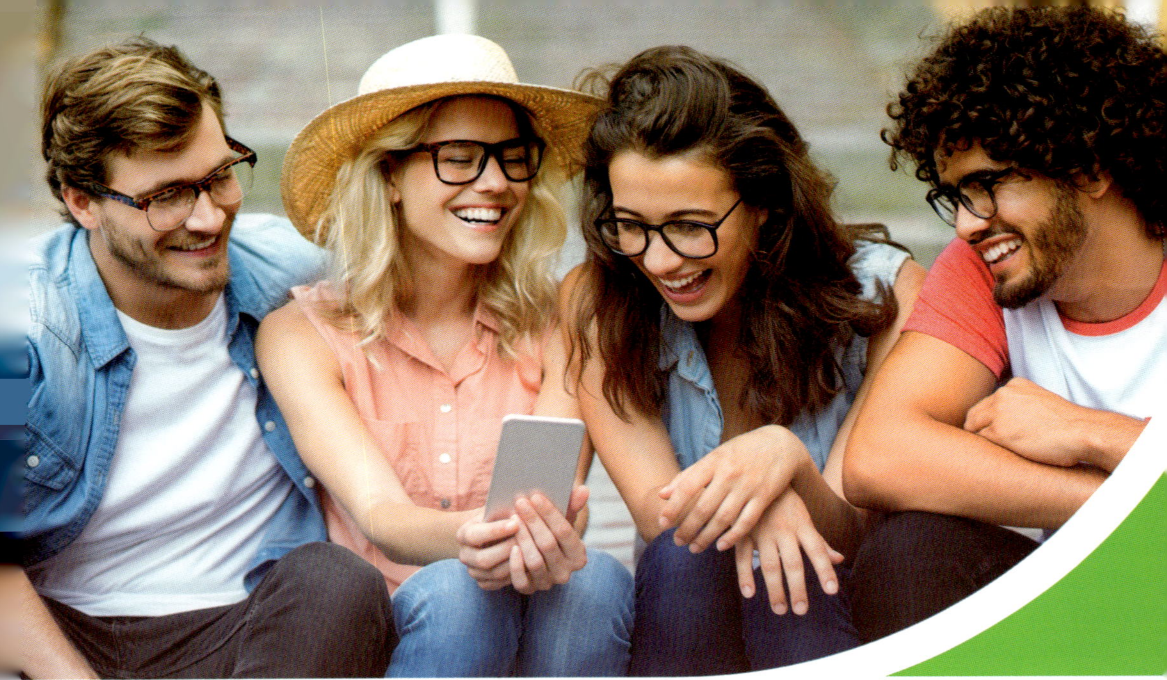

psychologist for help. The psychologist and Maya work on the problem through talk therapy.

After a while, Maya learns to **cope** with her social media problem. She goes out to dinner with her friends. And she doesn't photograph the food. She talks and laughs with her family. She enjoys her real social life instead of life on social media.

SOCIAL MEDIA: POSITIVES AND NEGATIVES

Social media has a positive side. Friends keep in contact. They make plans to do fun things in real life. People share laughs about funny pictures and jokes. Social media even offers the latest news.

But spending too much time on social media can become a problem. Problematic social media use negatively affects a person's life. Someone with a social media

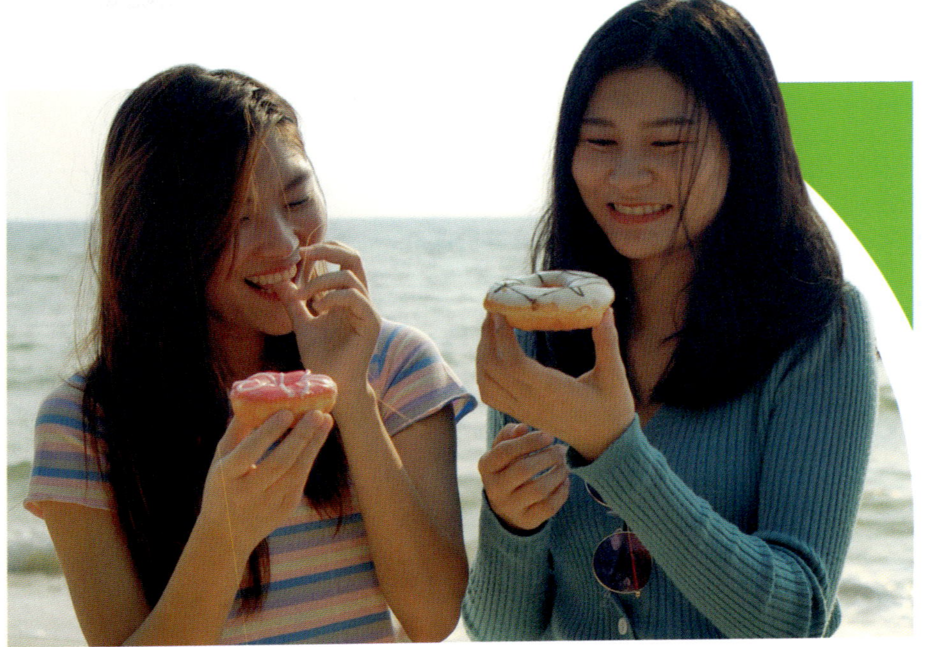

Sometimes it's best to enjoy the moment with friends without social media.

addiction might become physically and mentally unhealthy. Social media overuse interferes with real-life relationships. People facing this problem can get help from mental health professionals. They can learn to fully participate in real life. They can feel well again.

1

WHAT IS PROBLEMATIC SOCIAL MEDIA USE?

Social media includes websites or apps that let people interact. There are many types of social media. Facebook is one example. People write posts. They also share photos and videos. Facebook friends reply with comments. They can click the "like" button. The button has options for

reactions such as "love," "haha," or "wow."
They might also share others' posts.

Instagram is another example. People share photos and videos on Instagram. It lets followers comment on or like a post.

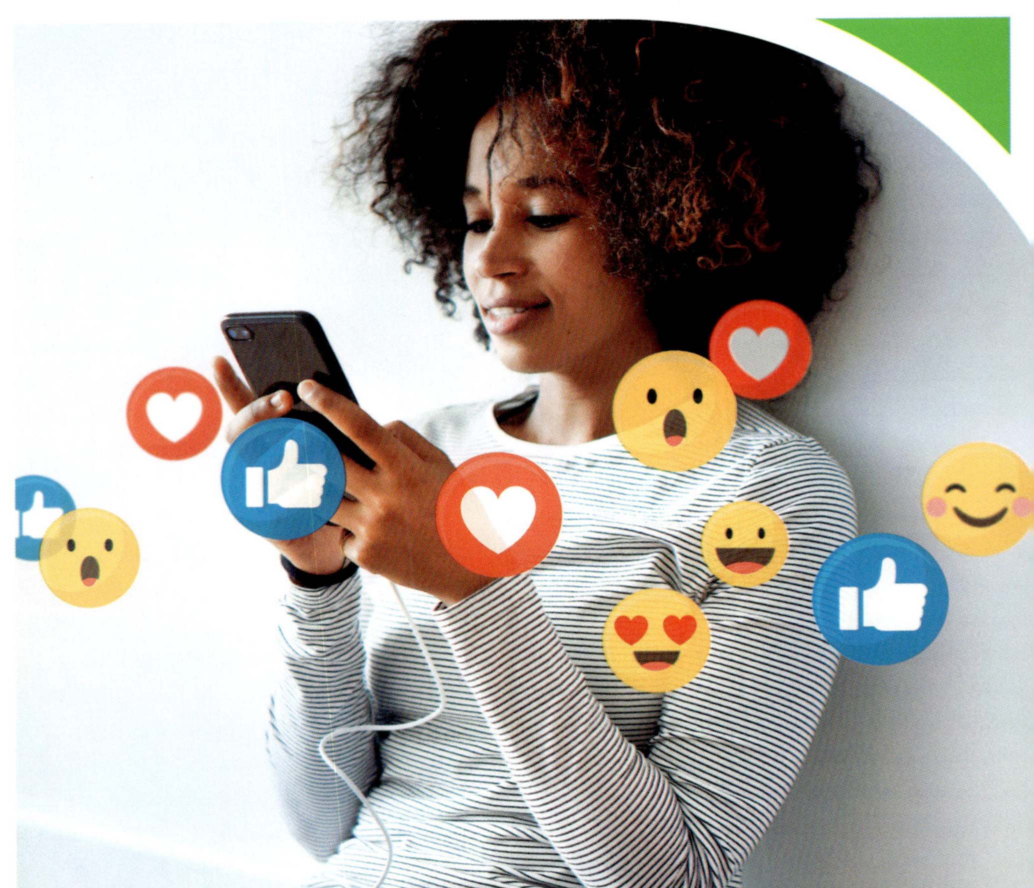

People who use Twitter write tweets.
Tweets are short text posts. They are limited
to a certain number of words. Twitter users
share photos and videos, too. Followers
can comment on a tweet, like it, or share it
with others.

Many people use the social media site
Reddit. This lets them connect with people
who have shared interests. The site offers
pages on everything from favorite TV shows
to crochet. People upvote or downvote
posts. Users are awarded points for the
upvotes they get. Snapchat is a popular
social media app. Its photos and videos

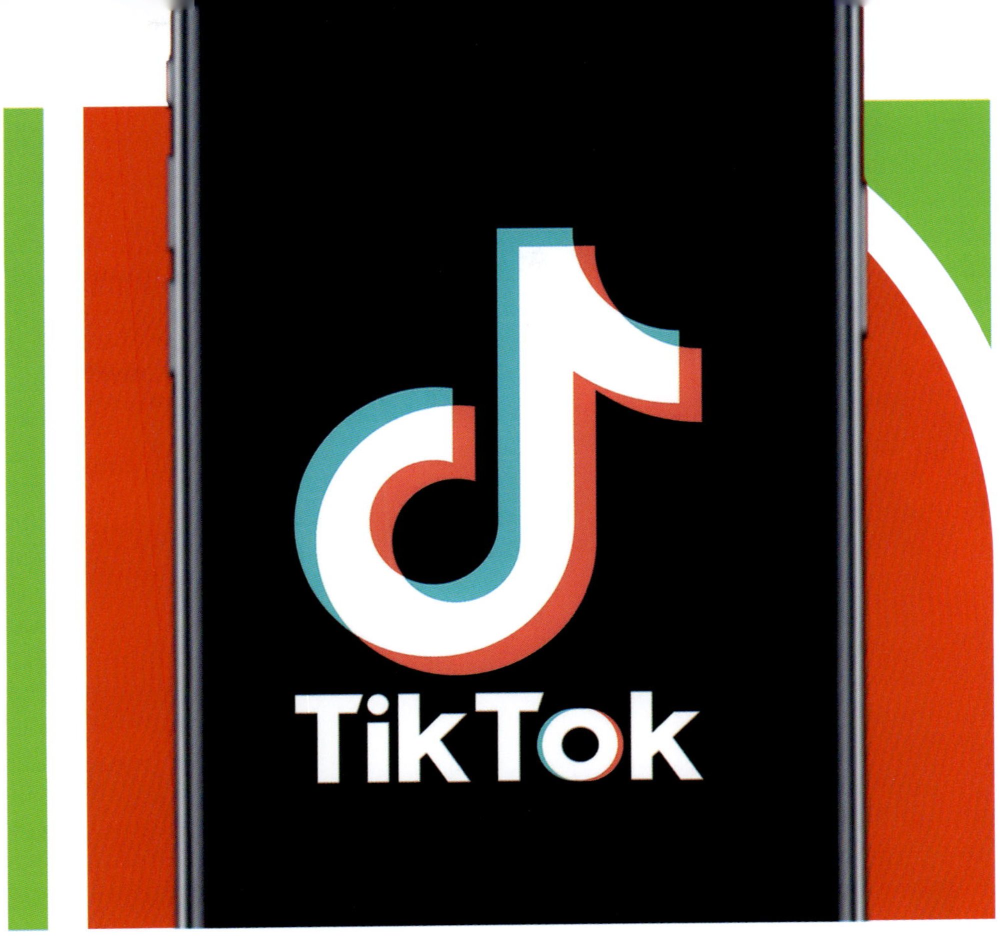

TikTok has more than 1 billion users worldwide.

disappear soon after they are shared. On

TikTok, users share short videos. Then

others respond to those videos. Even

multiplayer online games have social

interaction. They are a type of social media.

WHAT IS ADDICTION?

Social media can connect people. It can be fun. But some people spend too much time on it. It interferes with their lives. This is problematic social media use. Some people call this social media addiction. However, not everyone agrees with this term. The American Psychiatric Association (APA) defines addictions. The APA does not define social media overuse as an addiction.

The APA wrote the *Diagnostic and Statistical Manual of Mental Disorders, Fifth Edition* (*DSM-5*). Mental health professionals use this book to **diagnose** mental

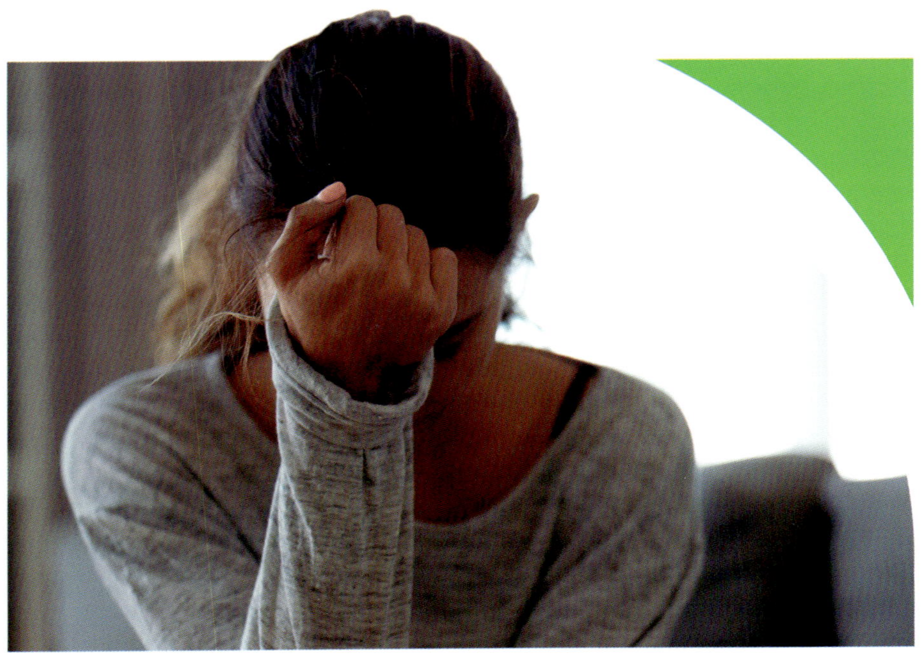

disorders. The *DSM-5* mentions addiction

to substances. These include alcohol,

nicotine, and other drugs.

Some people have substance addiction.

They keep using a substance even though

it harms them. The addiction causes

physical harm. It also causes mental harm.

These people crave the substance. If they stop using it, they feel unwell. The addiction disrupts their daily lives.

A behavioral addiction is something people do even though it harms them. The behavior does not involve substances. The APA explains, "Gambling disorder is the only behavioral addiction . . . identified in *DSM-5*."[1]

The *DSM-5* also discusses internet gaming disorder. The *DSM-5* says that it needs further study. It is not yet considered an addiction. Problematic social media use also needs more study.

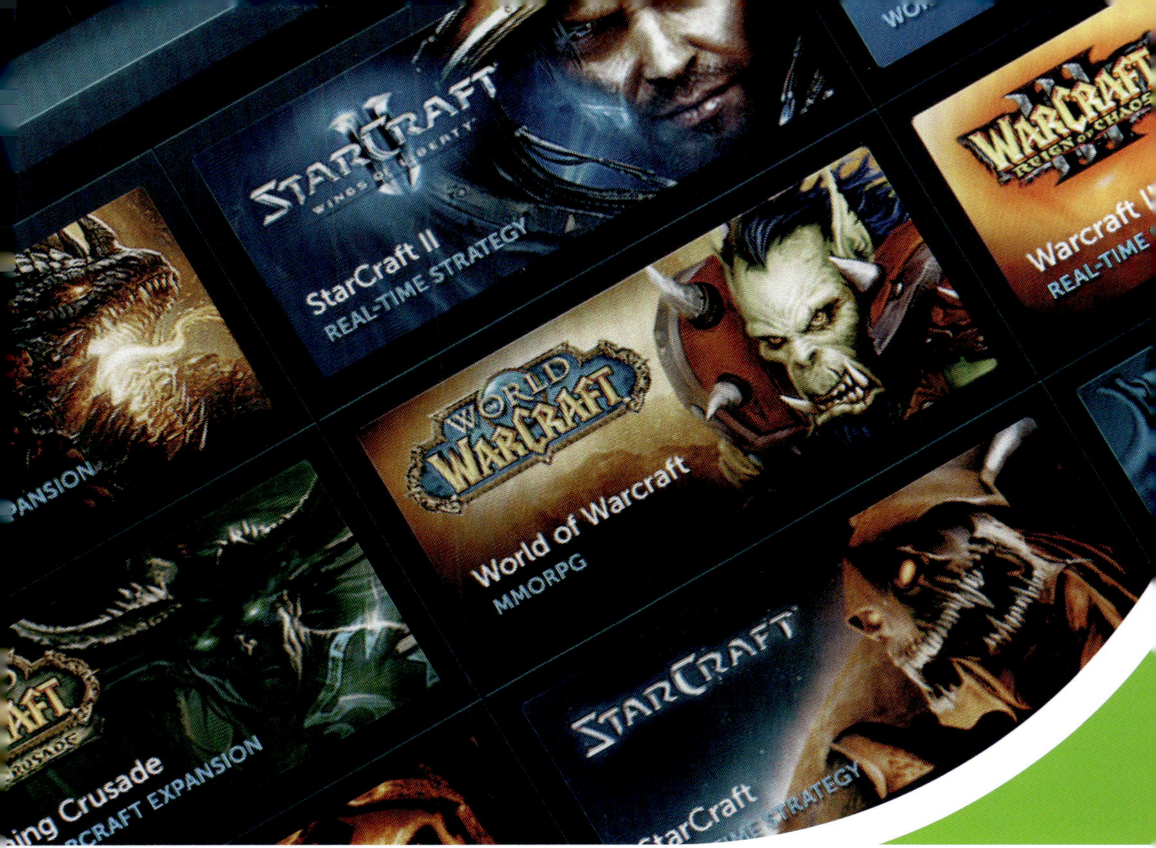

Millions of people play massively multiplayer online games such as World of Warcraft.

INTERNET GAMING DISORDER

Many experts consider multiplayer internet gaming to be social media. One example is *World of Warcraft*. This game has thousands of players. The players can interact. They build relationships that exist in and out of the game. Some people play online games too much.

The *DSM-5* proposes a new disorder. It is called internet gaming disorder. Understanding this disorder can help in understanding problematic social media use. The *DSM-5* suggests how to diagnose this disorder. The gaming must cause "significant impairment or distress" in many areas of a person's life.[2] The *DSM-5* lists nine symptoms. At least five of them must be present for one year. They are much like gambling disorder's symptoms.

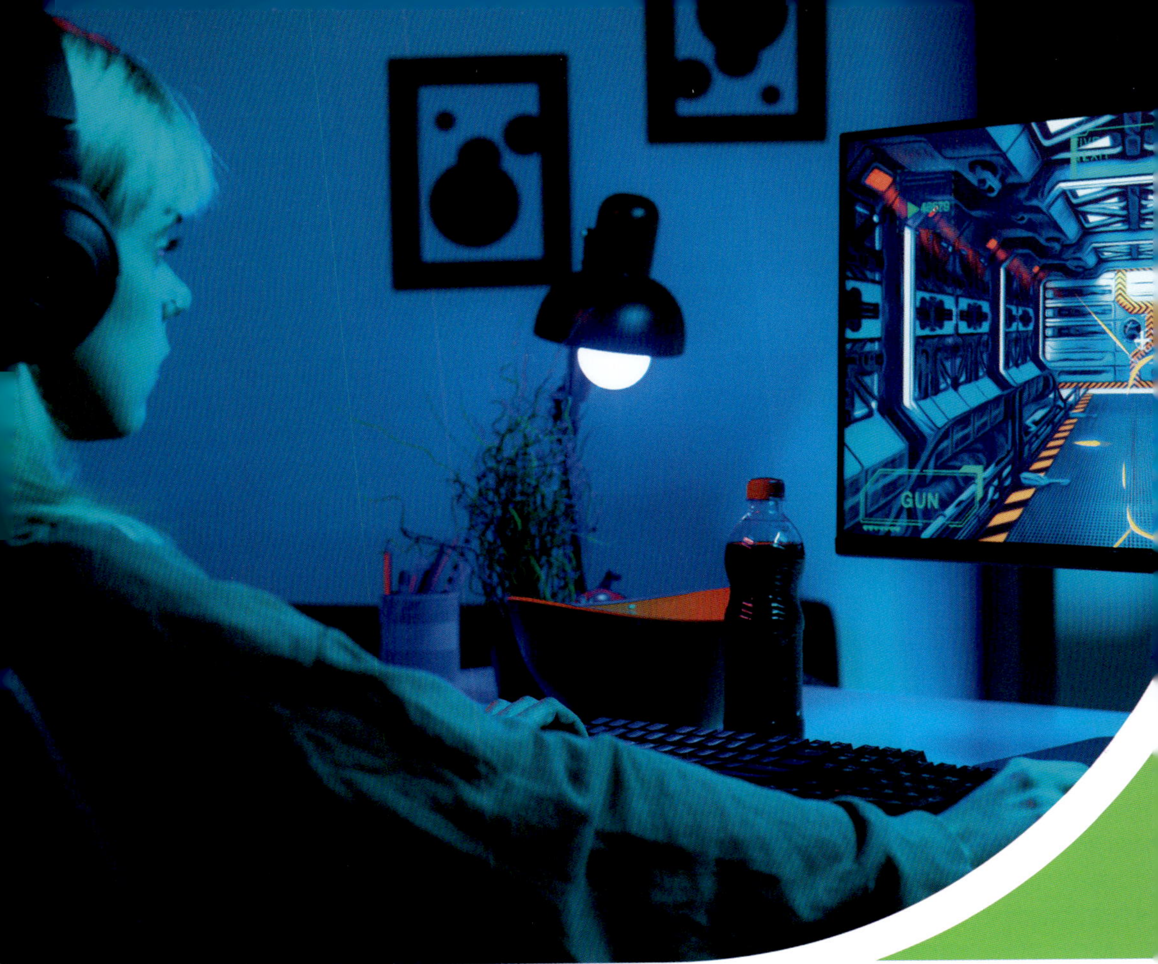

Someone with internet gaming disorder spends most of their available time gaming.

A person with internet gaming disorder constantly thinks about gaming. When he stops gaming, he experiences **withdrawal**. Withdrawal may include feelings of depression or anxiety. The person needs to game more and more to get the feeling he wants. This experience is called tolerance. The person is not successful when he tries to stop gaming.

Someone with a gaming problem chooses gaming over other activities. Gaming causes problems in his life. But he won't stop playing. He lies to others about the time he spends gaming. He uses gaming to deal with negative feelings. And finally, he risks his job or relationships. He puts gaming first.

SOCIAL NETWORKING ADDICTION

Psychologist Mark D. Griffiths studies behavior related to social networking sites (SNSs). SNSs are forms of social media. Griffiths says that SNSs are where people interact with real-life friends online. People can also meet others with the same interests.

ATTENTION EQUALS CARING

James P. Steyer wrote the book *Talking Back to Facebook*. Steyer says that people show they care by paying attention. Someone who is always on social media sends the opposite message. For example, a person scrolls social media during family night. She is not showing her family she cares about them.

Griffiths offers six markers of SNS addiction. First, the addicted person constantly thinks about social sites. Second, the person's mood changes when using those sites. Third, she develops a tolerance. She needs to spend more time on the sites to feel the same effects.

Fourth, the person with SNS addiction has withdrawal symptoms. Fifth, she has conflicts with herself or other people. Sixth, she **relapses**. She tries to stop. But she returns to the addictive behavior. Many experts use Griffiths's six markers when they discuss social media addiction.

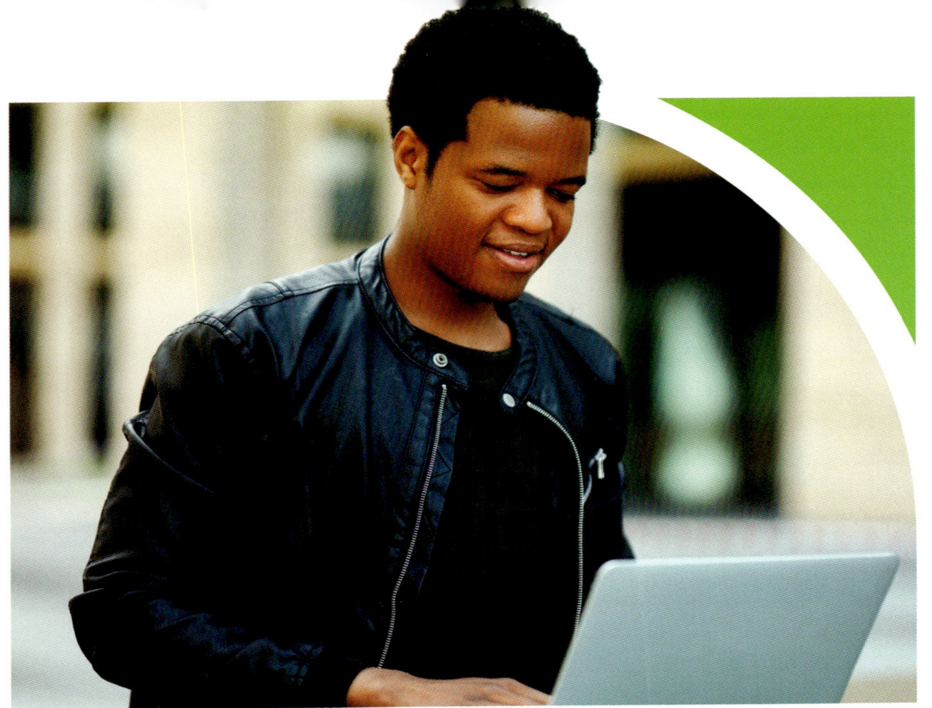

People may experience mood changes when using social media. These mood changes can influence addiction.

HOW COMMON IS PROBLEMATIC SOCIAL MEDIA USE?

Fanni Bányai is a researcher. In 2015, she

and other researchers studied 5,961 teens

and their social media use. The study

found that 4.5 percent of the teens were

TEENS' FAVORITE SOCIAL MEDIA SERVICES

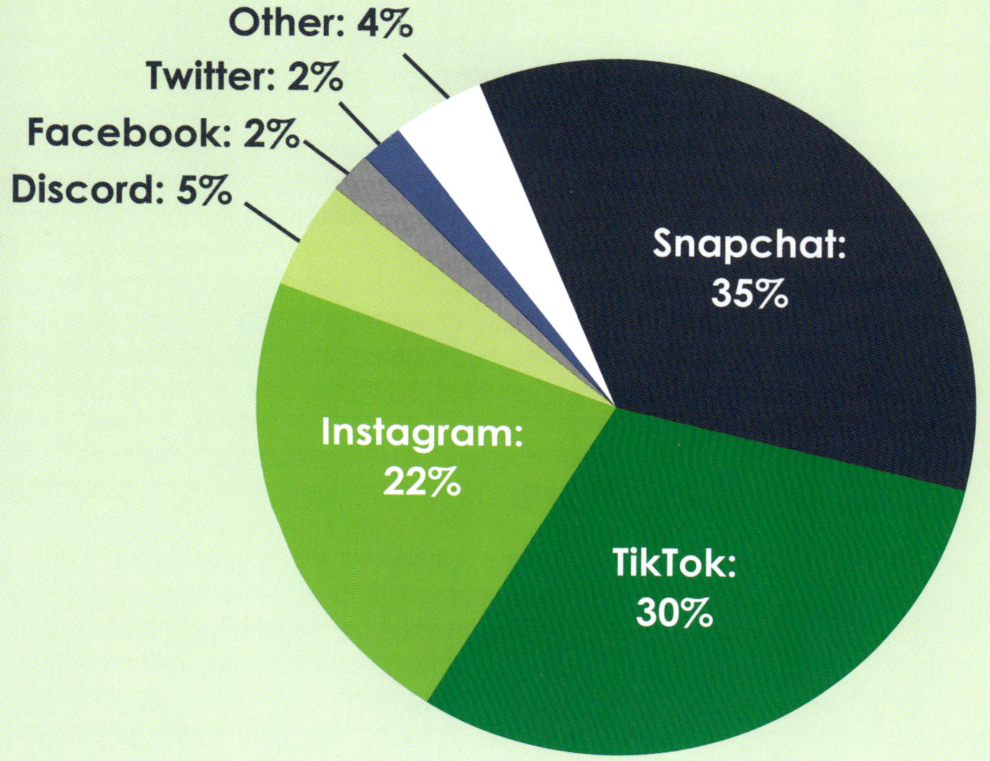

Source: "Taking Stock with Teens: 21 Years of Researching US Teens GenZ Insights," Piper Sandler, Fall 2021. www.pipersandler.com.

A 2021 survey asked teens what their favorite social media sites were. This chart shows how they responded. The surveyed teens spent about four hours a day on social media.

at risk for problematic social media use.
The researchers also found that there were
more teenage girls than boys in the at-risk
group. Other studies suggest that internet
gaming problems are more common
among boys than girls. Researchers Daria
Kuss and Griffiths say that more studies are
needed. These studies should explore the
demographics of social media addiction.

Pew Research Center surveyed teens in
2018. It asked about their social media use.
Twenty-four percent of teens thought social
media negatively affected them. They said it
led to bullying. It also harmed relationships.

2

THE SCIENCE OF SOCIAL MEDIA ADDICTION

The brain plays an important part in addiction. The brain has about 86 billion neurons. Neurons are nerve cells. They communicate with each other. They do this with electric and chemical signals. The chemicals that send messages between neurons are called neurotransmitters.

Dopamine is a neurotransmitter. It is part of the brain's reward system. For example, dopamine is released in the brain when someone eats a tasty chocolate. The person feels rewarded. He feels good.

The substantia nigra (highlighted) is one of the places in the brain that produces dopamine.

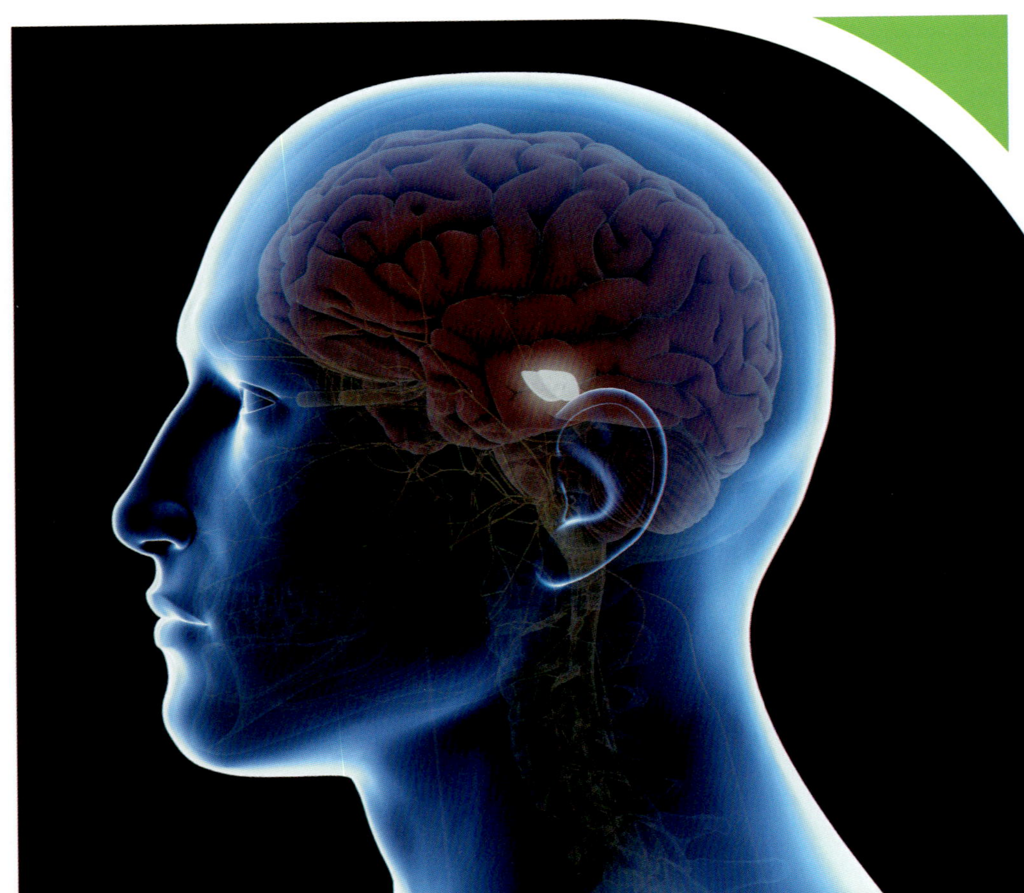

He will want to eat the chocolate again.

Dopamine also is released when people

have positive social contact. This applies to

positive interactions on social media.

Dopamine is linked to addiction.

Dopamine encourages people to repeat

actions that feel good. Someone with

an addiction repeats the action even if it

causes her harm.

SOCIAL MEDIA AND BEHAVIOR

The first president of Facebook was Sean

Parker. He said the purpose of Facebook

is to take as much of a user's time and

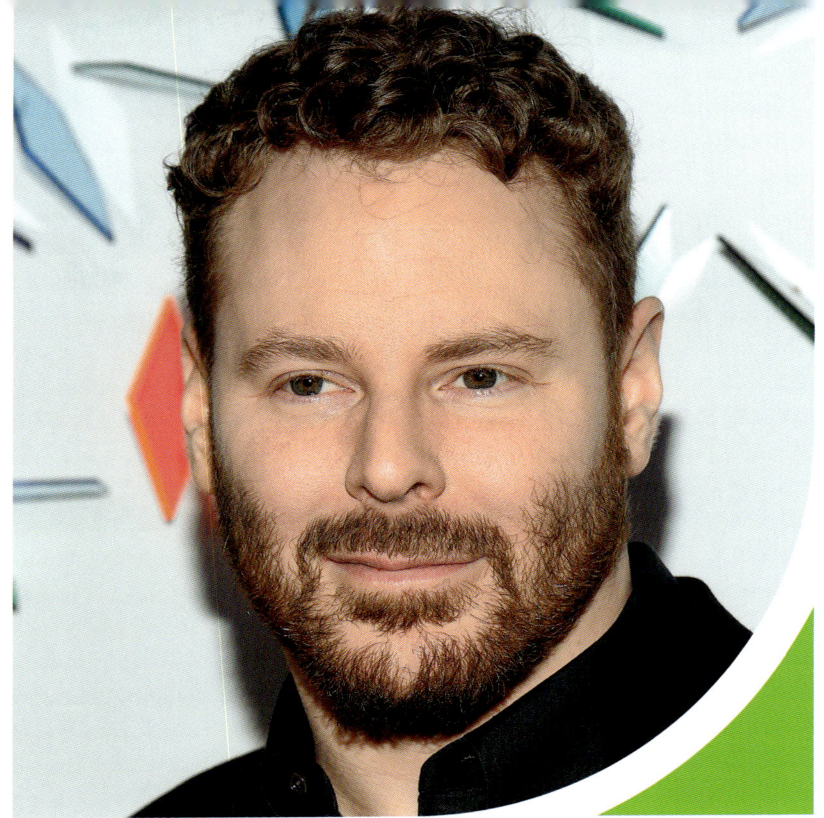

Sean Parker joined Facebook in 2004. He continued to influence the company after he left a year later.

attention as possible. Facebook does

this with positive social rewards. A like

releases dopamine in a user's brain. This

reward keeps the person coming back

to Facebook.

Learning by adding a reward is called positive reinforcement. Learning by taking away something undesirable is called negative reinforcement. A person who uses social media experiences positive reinforcement. She is rewarded with likes or

PAVLOV'S DOGS AND SOCIAL MEDIA NOTIFICATIONS

Scientist Ivan Pavlov studied dogs. When he fed them, he played a clicking sound. At first, the dogs' mouths watered because of the food. But over time, the dogs' mouths watered when they heard the sound alone. Social media users show similar behavior. They check social media when they hear a notification sound.

kind comments. She learns to keep coming back for more rewards.

Another person scrolls social media because he feels stressed. He learns to use it to escape negative experiences. His actions are the result of negative reinforcement.

How often positive reinforcement is given also affects behavior. People repeat actions more if they do not know when they will be rewarded. Positive rewards on social media are unpredictable. This is why users check the sites or apps often.

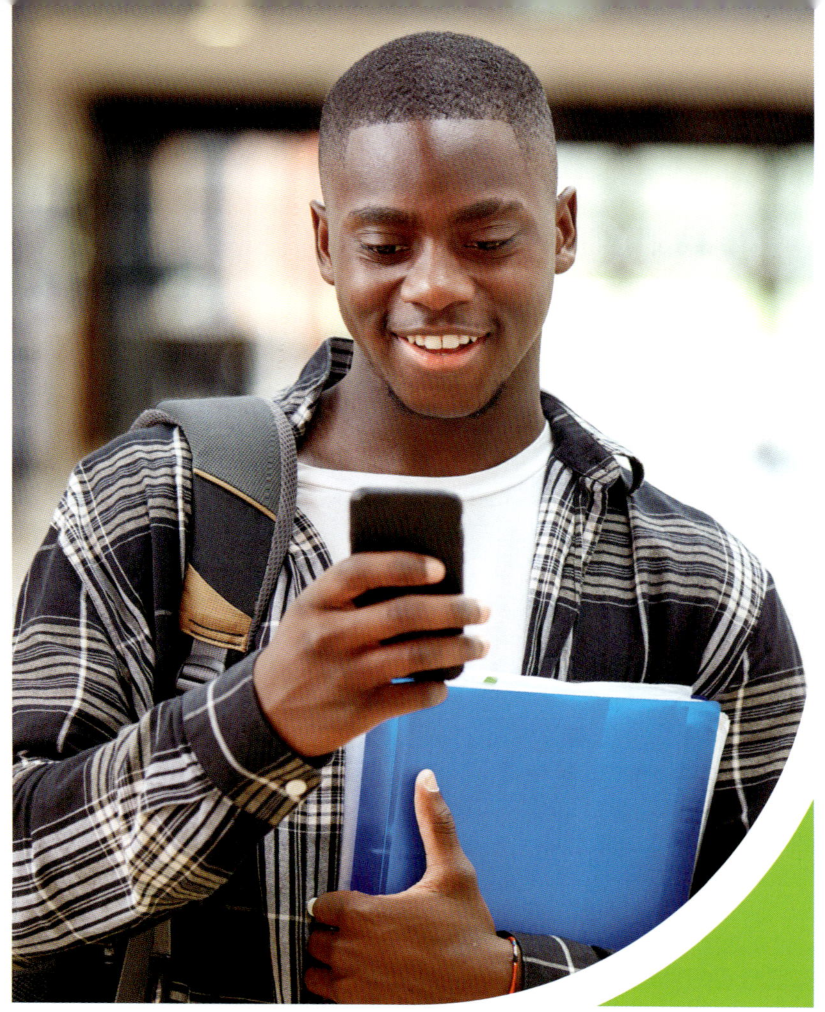

Teens' brains send reward signals when the teens see that their photos have many likes.

ALGORITHMS AND ADDICTION

Social media uses computer **algorithms**.

These algorithms change what a user sees.

The algorithms gather information about the user's behavior, such as her interests. Then the algorithms adjust her feed.

Professors Vikram R. Bhargava and Manuel Velasquez wrote about social media addiction. They talked about algorithms. The algorithms "change the website itself to increase its own addictive potential for each particular user."[3]

THE ENDLESS SCROLL

Most social media sites or apps do not require users to reload at the bottom of a page. New content loads automatically. There are no cues to stop. So users continue to scroll. Social media users often lose track of time during endless scrolling.

3
THE EFFECTS OF PROBLEMATIC SOCIAL MEDIA USE

Social media overuse often negatively affects a person's life. Dar Meshi and Morgan Ellithorpe are researchers. They found that problematic social media use was related to increased depression. It was also linked to more anxiety and social **isolation**.

DEPRESSION AND ANXIETY

Depression is a mental health disorder. A person with depression might feel extremely sad. He might lack energy and be tired. He might not like doing things he used to enjoy.

People who are isolated often feel lonely or depressed.

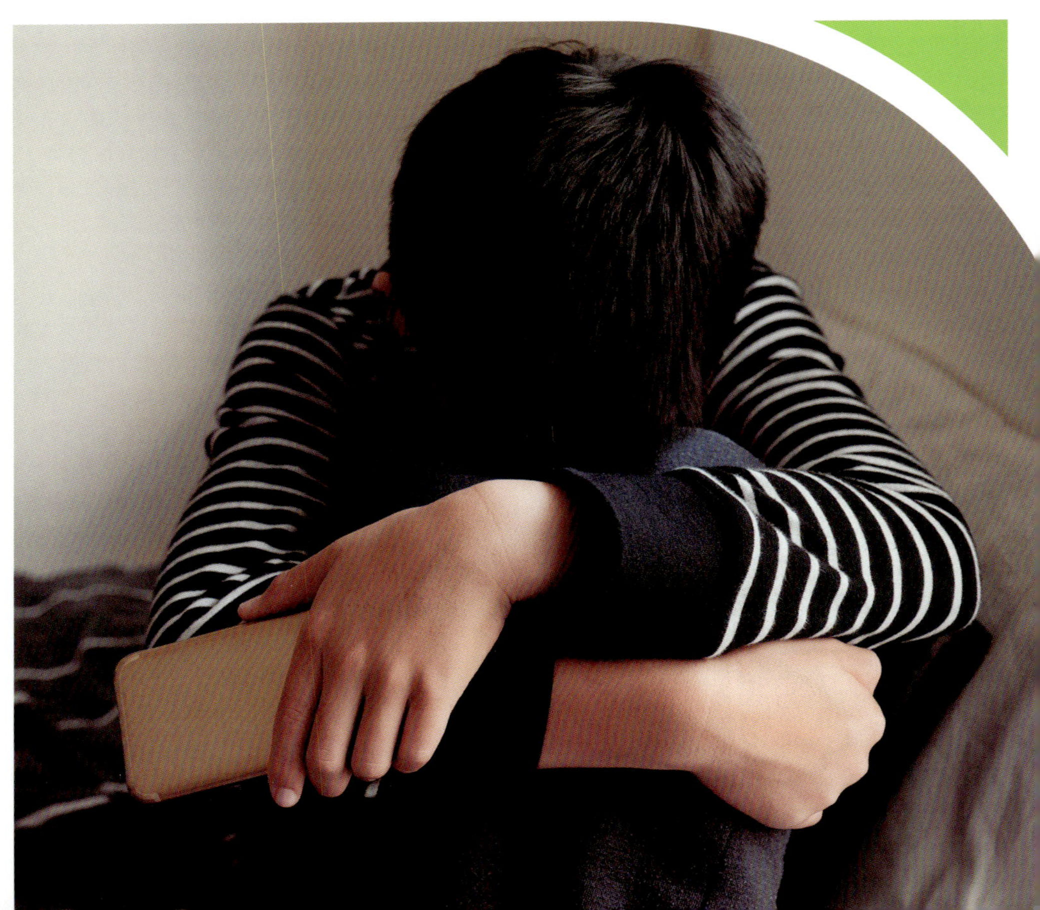

Depression can also affect someone's sleeping and eating.

A person with anxiety might feel on edge. She is easily bothered. She might be constantly worried. She gets poor sleep.

People often have both problematic social media use and mental health disorders. But this does not prove that social media addiction causes these disorders. People with depression or anxiety may be more likely to overuse social media. Further research is needed to understand the link between social media and mental health.

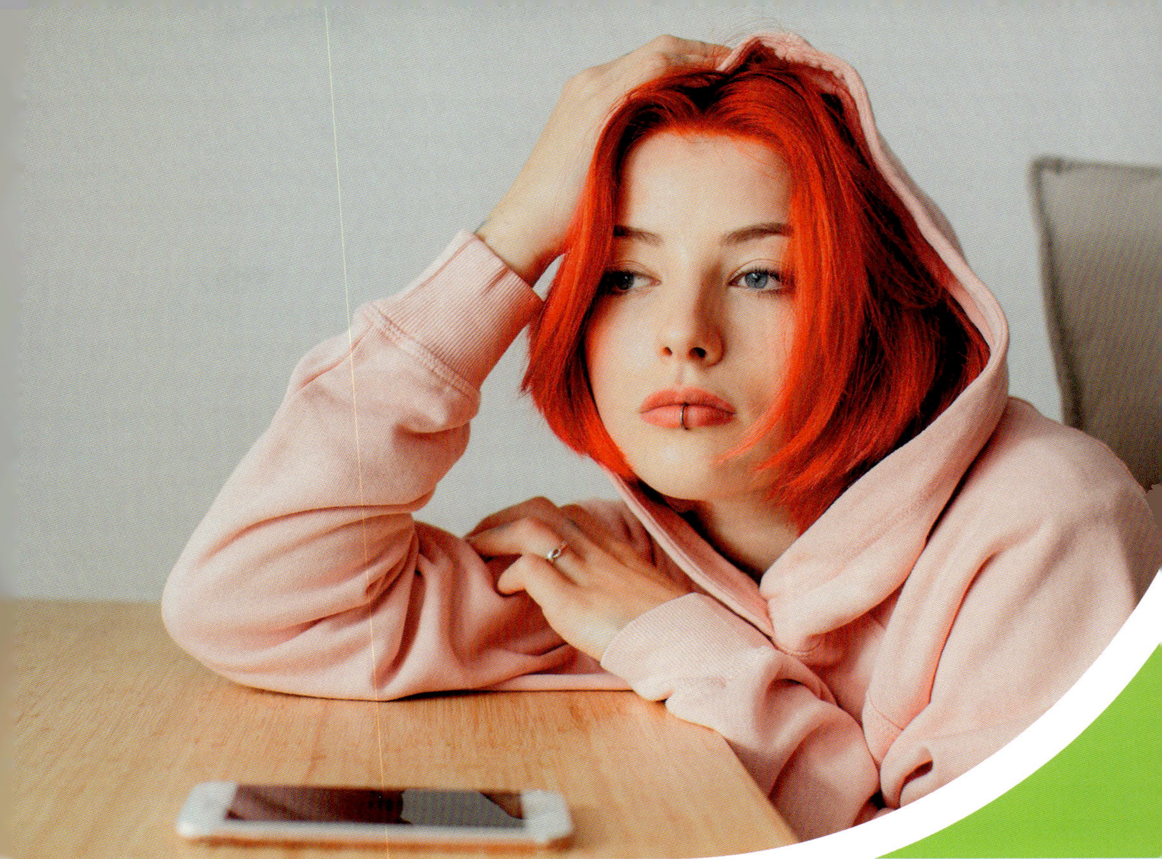

Studies suggest that people who often use social media tend to be less happy with life.

Problematic social media use can affect physical health. Russell Viner and fellow researchers studied these effects. They found that social media overuse can disrupt activities. Two examples are exercise and sleep. A lack of exercise can lead to physical health problems.

People may choose to scroll social media instead of walking or biking. They miss out on the benefits of exercise. Regular exercise protects against heart disease and diabetes. It lowers blood pressure. It also improves sleep. Exercise releases brain chemicals called endorphins. They make the person exercising feel good.

Exercise even improves mental health. Dr. Michael Craig Miller is an assistant professor of psychiatry. He explains that exercise helps neurons grow in the brain.

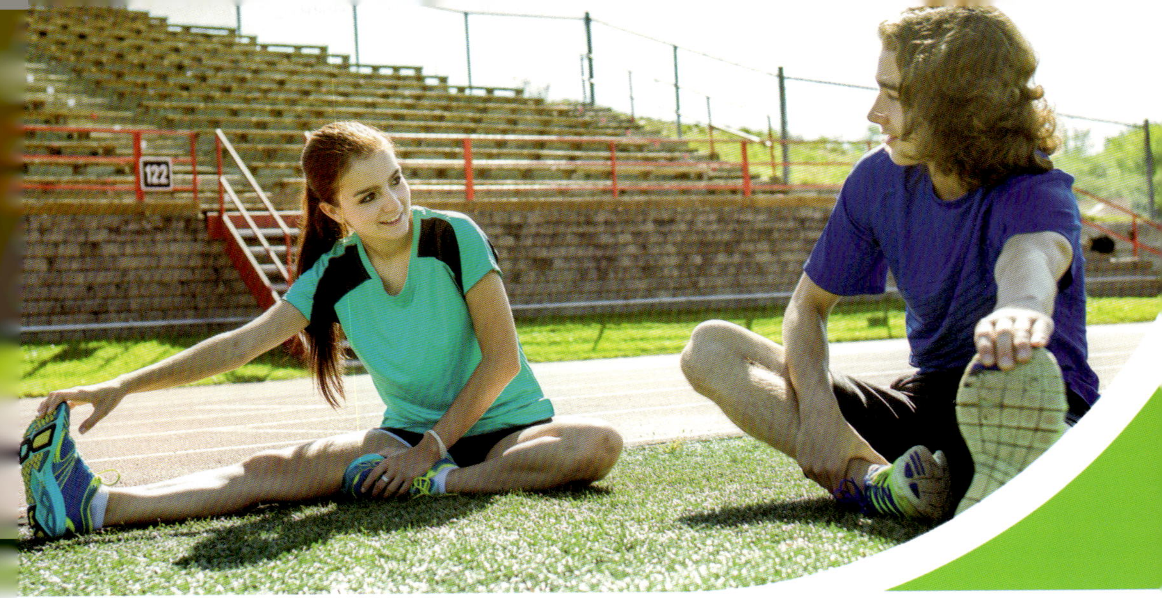

This relieves depression. Exercise also reduces anxiety. It takes a person's focus off worries. It relaxes tense muscles.

Social media overuse might keep someone from sleeping well. Social media users often take devices into their bedrooms. They surf social media late into the night. They do not get enough sleep.

Smartphones and computers give off blue light. This light suppresses melatonin. Melatonin is a chemical in the body. It tells the body when to sleep.

A lack of sleep can be bad for physical and mental health. People are more likely to become physically ill without enough sleep. Losing sleep can negatively affect a person's mood. It can increase stress levels. People may have trouble concentrating, too.

RELATIONSHIPS

People who overuse social media often lose touch with their real-life friends and

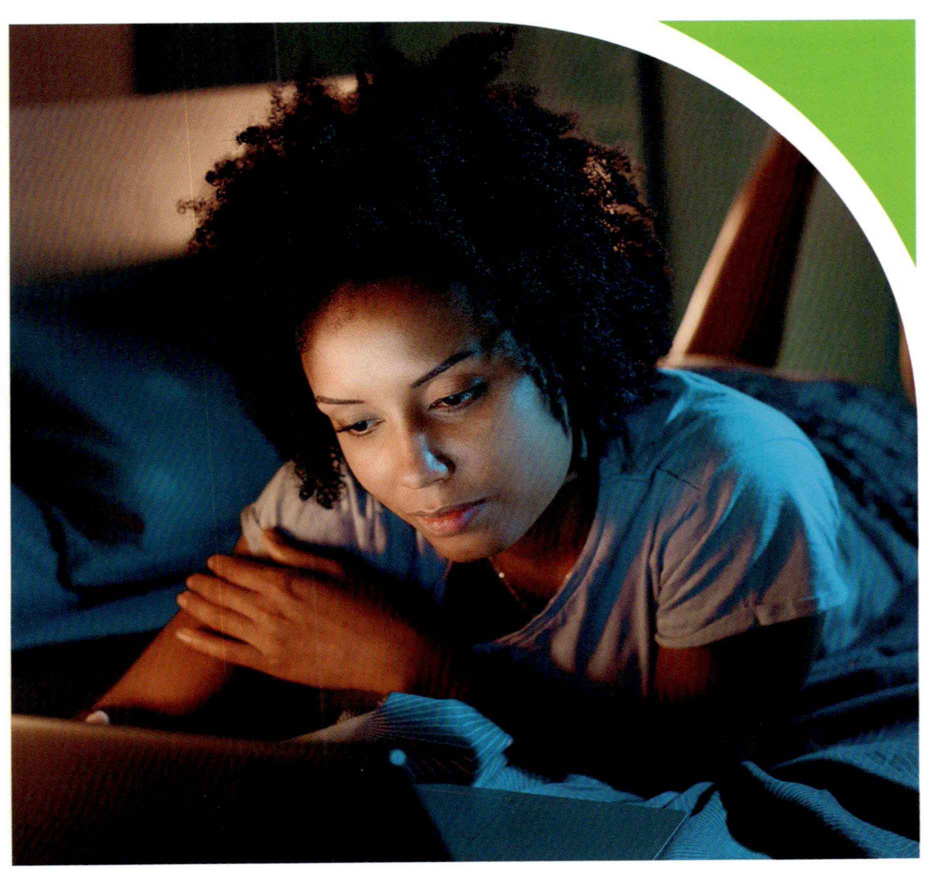

family. Zach Lee led a 2012 study. He

found that online socializing increased

social separation in real life. Some people

choose to engage most with social media

friends and followers. They miss out on relationships with people in real life. This leads to isolation and loneliness.

Sherry Turkle is a professor of social studies. She studies science and technology. She has observed families sitting at the kitchen table. They all are focused on social media. They ignore each other. Turkle describes this behavior as "being alone together."[4] She worries that so many people using social media could lead to increased isolation.

Experts worry that social media overuse affects young people's ability to communicate in person. Young people decide to private message, comment, and text. They do this instead of talking face-to-face. Without in-person conversation, they don't learn to understand communication cues. These cues include body language, facial expressions, and tone

SOCIAL MEDIA AND SCHOOLWORK

Social media may distract from homework. A person with social media addiction may skip homework to spend time online. He scrolls on social media for hours. Then, there isn't time to do a good job on schoolwork. Avoiding homework often causes grades to fall.

of voice. Young people may be slowly losing the art of making conversation.

Experts are also concerned about people having less empathy. Empathy is the ability to understand what another person feels. On social media, a person doesn't see the effect her posts and comments have on others. It is easy to ignore people's feelings online. She may have less empathy.

For example, someone says something mean to another in person. She watches him frown. She sees his tears fall. She knows she hurt his feelings. She feels bad. If she says something mean on social

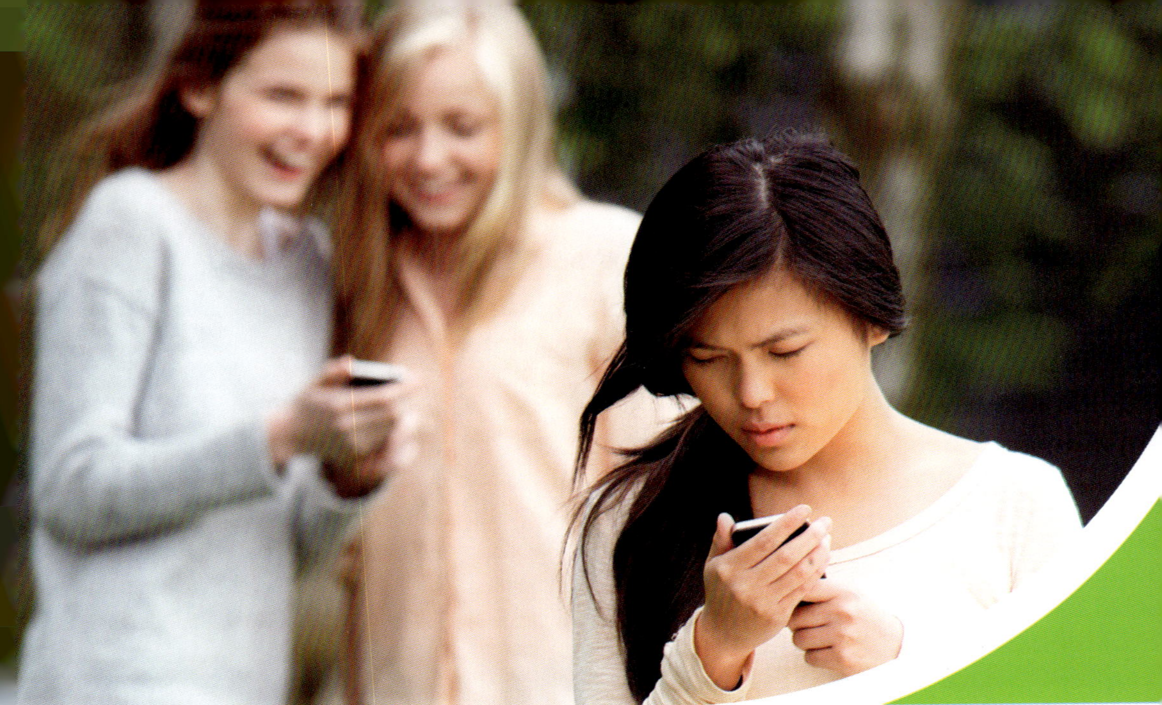

media, she won't see he is hurt. She might

not feel empathy for him.

SELF-ESTEEM

Alyssa Saiphoo and fellow researchers

looked at how social media use impacts

self-esteem. Self-esteem is how much a

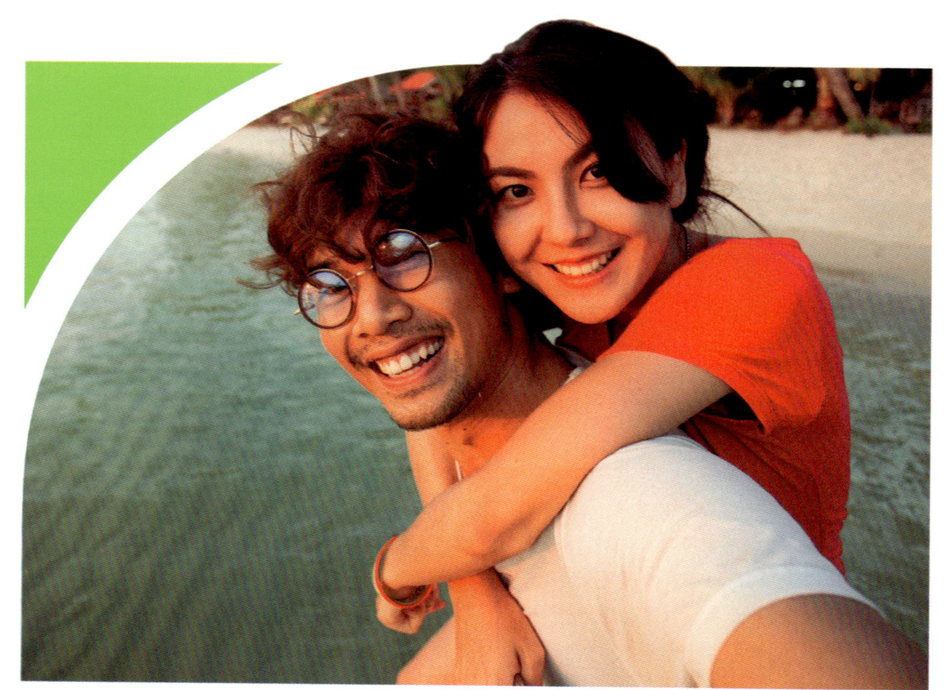

person values herself. Saiphoo found that greater use of social media is associated with lower levels of self-esteem.

People who overuse social media might have low self-esteem because they compare themselves to others. They see friends posting about fun trips or parties.

Then they feel bad about themselves.

Dr. Michelle Quilter is a psychologist. She explains, "It's comparing the way you feel inside to other people's outsides."[5] And the "outsides" that people post are mostly the positives. They don't write about the English test they failed or their fights with siblings.

THE CYCLE OF NEGATIVE SOCIAL MEDIA USE

Some people go onto social media when they feel stressed or upset. But more social media use can hurt their self-esteem. This may worsen their mood. Then they use social media more. They hope it will help them feel better. But it actually makes them feel worse.

4
TREATING PROBLEMATIC SOCIAL MEDIA USE

People with problematic social media use have hope. There are many treatments available. Mental health professionals can help. These include psychiatrists, psychologists, and social workers.

SEEKING TREATMENT

Doctors often suggest having a physical exam before seeking mental health treatment. A physical exam checks for any medical issues that could cause symptoms. For example, thyroid problems

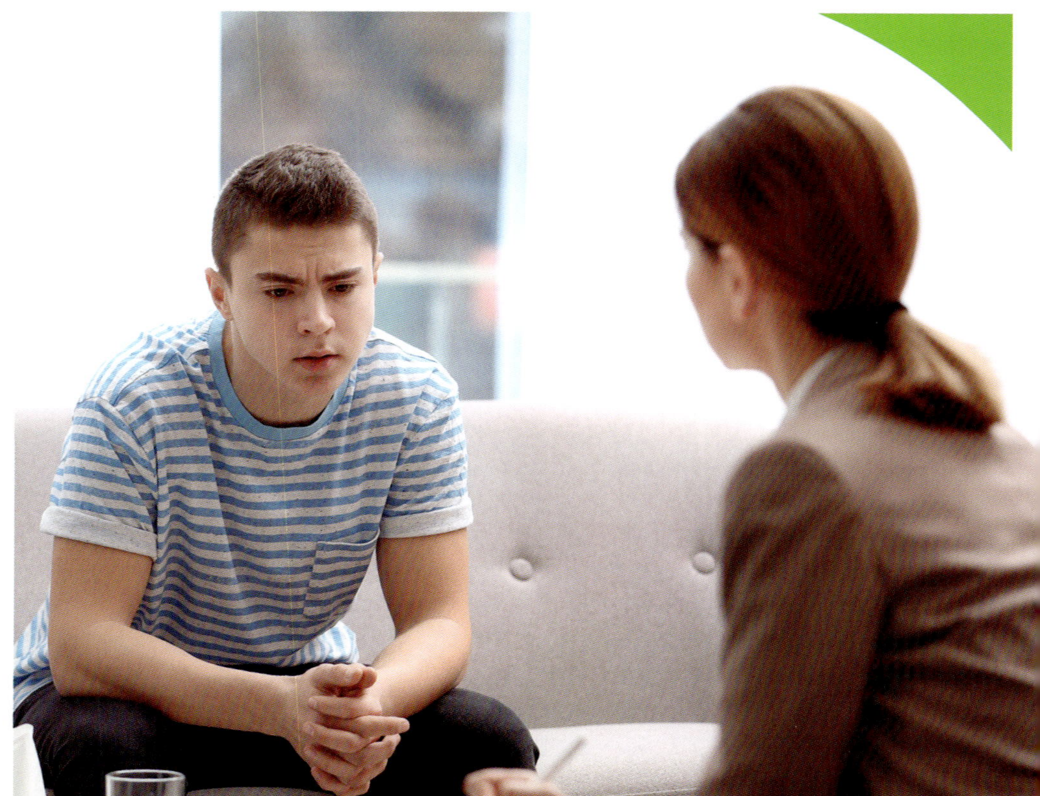

Psychologists can help people with social media addiction.

can cause depression. Physical issues are addressed first. Then the person can seek mental health treatment.

THERAPY

Talk therapy is a great treatment option for social media overuse. With talk therapy, patients speak one-on-one with mental health professionals.

Cognitive behavioral therapy (CBT) is a type of talk therapy. It can effectively treat problematic social media use. CBT helps change a person's behavior and thoughts. When behavior changes, so do thoughts.

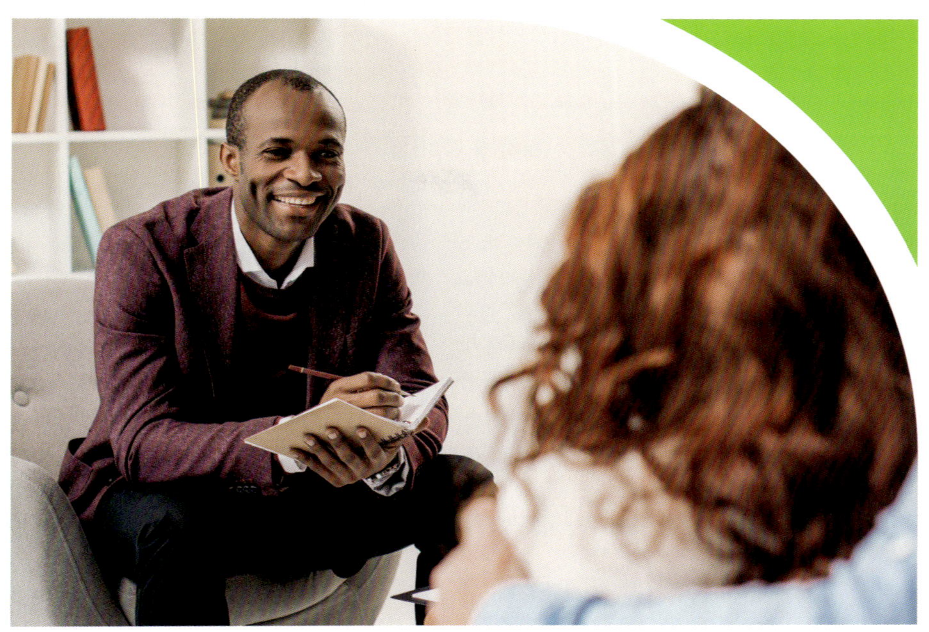

Sometimes people with social media addiction have other mental health disorders. Psychiatrists can help treat these.

And when thoughts change, so does behavior. CBT is a short-term treatment. It usually lasts around twelve weeks. The patient is often given homework.

Dialectical behavior therapy (DBT) is another treatment. Quilter says that DBT combines CBT and mindfulness. She says that mindfulness is being focused on the present without judgment. For example, a person practicing mindfulness might hike in the woods. She focuses on her breathing and the sounds around her. Quilter says, "Social media is a mindless activity. Replace it with mindfulness."[6]

PRACTICAL SOLUTIONS

There are things a person with problematic social media use can do to help himself. Dr. Meghan Miller is the director of health education at the Floating Hospital. She says

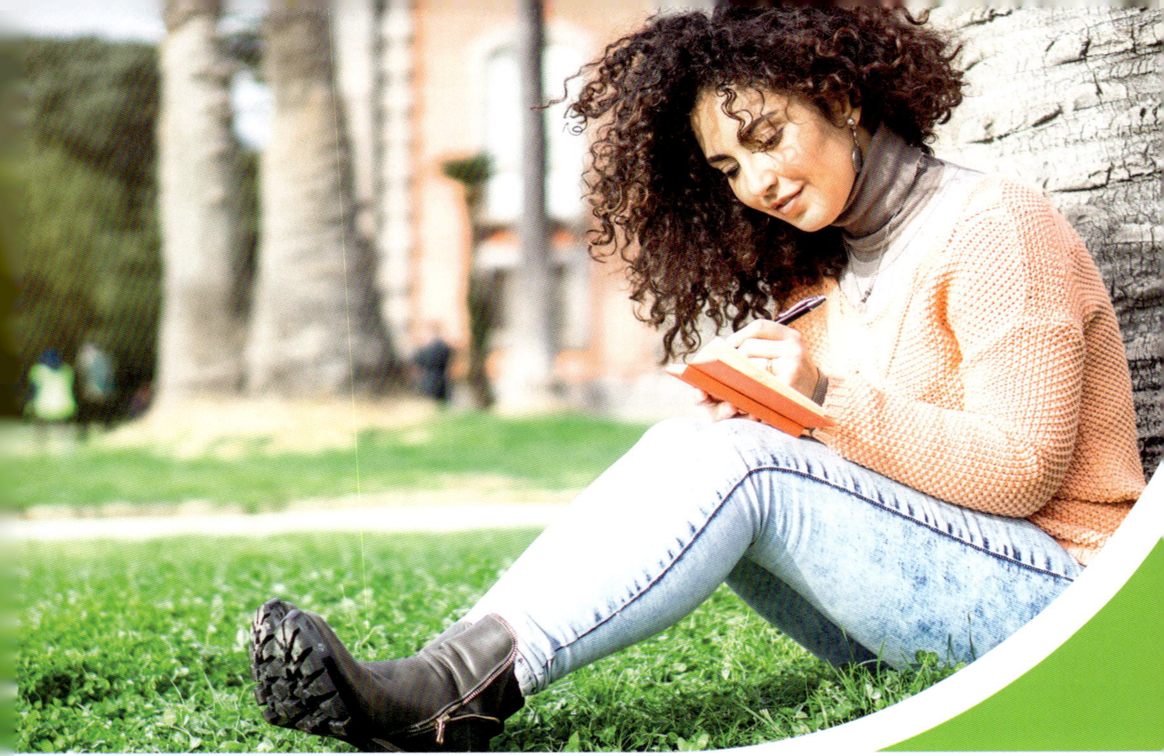

that boredom can lead to social media overuse. She suggests doing fun things with people in real life. A person could take a dance class or join a club.

There are practical ways to stay off social media. A person can move the smartphone or computer to a different room. He is less likely to mindlessly surf social media if he needs to move to do it. School psychologist Jennifer Obrizok suggests charging the device in a parent's room. Miller says to set a timer. Then get off social media when it sounds.

12-STEP PROGRAMS FOR SOCIAL MEDIA ADDICTION

A person with social media addiction might attend a 12-step program. People with addiction meet together. They help each other cope. People work the twelve steps to change their behavior and to lead more positive lives.

Technology can be useful in limiting social media use. For example, turn off notifications. Some social media sites and apps have timer features. These might close the app when time runs out. A person can also block certain sites and apps.

Problematic social media use can cause many difficulties in a person's life. It is linked to physical and mental health disorders. Social media overuse can harm relationships and lead to loneliness. But there are effective treatments available. They offer help to those with social media addiction.

GLOSSARY

algorithms

steps computer programs use to accomplish a task

cope

to deal with a difficult situation well

demographics

characteristics of a population, such as age or gender

diagnose

to determine what a physical or mental health issue is by looking at its effects

isolation

the state of being separate from other people

relapses

returns to doing something after having tried to stop

withdrawal

psychological and physical symptoms that occur when an addictive substance or behavior is taken away

SOURCE NOTES

CHAPTER ONE: WHAT IS PROBLEMATIC SOCIAL MEDIA USE?

1. "Internet Gaming," *American Psychiatric Association*, June 2018. www.psychiatry.org

2. Quoted in "Internet Gaming."

CHAPTER TWO: THE SCIENCE OF SOCIAL MEDIA ADDICTION

3. Vikram R. Bhargava and Manuel Velasquez, "Ethics of the Attention Economy: The Problem of Social Media Addiction," *Business Ethics Quarterly*, July 2021, p. 334.

CHAPTER THREE: THE EFFECTS OF PROBLEMATIC SOCIAL MEDIA USE

4. Sherry Turkle, "Connected, but Alone?" *TED*, February 2012. www.ted.com.

5. Michelle Quilter, PsyD, Personal interview, November 28, 2021.

CHAPTER FOUR: TREATING PROBLEMATIC SOCIAL MEDIA USE

6. Michelle Quilter, PsyD, Personal interview, November 28, 2021.

FOR FURTHER RESEARCH

BOOKS

Tammy Gagne, *Developing Relationship Skills*. San Diego, CA: BrightPoint Press, 2023.

Duchess Harris and Elisabeth Herschbach, *Your Personalized Internet*. Minneapolis, MN: Abdo, 2018.

Kizzi Roberts, *Gaming Addiction*. San Diego, CA: BrightPoint Press, 2023.

INTERNET SOURCES

Trevor Haynes, "Dopamine, Smartphones & You: A Battle for Your Time," *Science in the News: Harvard University*, May 1, 2018. https://sitn.hms.harvard.edu.

"Internet Gaming," *American Psychiatric Association*, June 2018. www.psychiatry.org.

Sherry Turkle, "Connected, but Alone?" *TED*, 2012. www.ted.com.

WEBSITES

American Psychiatric Association
www.psychiatry.org

The American Psychiatric Association is a professional organization of psychiatrists. This website has reliable information about gaming disorder, addiction, depression, and anxiety.

National Alliance on Mental Illness (NAMI)
https://nami.org

NAMI is a mental health organization that helps those with mental illness. The website contains information on mental health disorders and treatment.

National Institute of Mental Health
www.nimh.nih.gov

This is the official website of the National Institute of Mental Health. The institute does mental health research. Its website provides current information about addiction and other mental health disorders.

INDEX

ABOUT THE AUTHOR

Marie-Therese Miller, PhD, writes nonfiction books for children and teens. Her most recent books include *Handling Depression, Teens and Cyberbullying*, and *Dealing with Psychotic Disorders*. Miller earned a PhD in English from St. John's University. Her academic focus was James Thurber and humor. She teaches Children's and Young Adult Literature at Marist College. Miller and her husband, John, have five children and a grandson.